Thanks to all who encouraged, inspired and supported my writing through the years.

To readers – I hope you find this short book to be useful in helping you or a loved one learn about, manage, live with being bipolar. I have updated this book and added some information I believe is helpful.

ISBN: 9781703605440

Any references to historical events, real people, or real places are used fictitiously. Names, characters, and places are products of the author's imagination.

Cover design by: Colleen Hurst

Second Printing 2020

While I have consulted with therapists and other individuals who have bipolar; this book is not a medical paper; it isn't written by a medical professional, and isn't a diagnosis, nor a diagnostic tool.

My purpose is only to put information out there that I learned in the course of my treatment, that someone else might relate to or even find helpful. My experiences may differ from others; as bipolar doesn't affect everyone the same way. All opinions and comments are based on my own experiences or conversations I have had with others; and may not apply to someone else with bipolar.

This is a book about having Bipolar Disorder: what it means, what it is, what it isn't, and how I learned to manage it. This has been written by someone who is bipolar; who was misdiagnosed three times before being correctly diagnosed. To treat something successfully, you have to first be diagnosed correctly.

I have been living with Bipolar Disorder; and, have been managing it with varying degrees of success since 2003. I want to share what I have learned with others in hopes that it will help them as they deal with it – whether they are in the early stages of being diagnosed, or already under treatment for years.

This book is intentionally relatively short because; having bipolar, I know that people who have Bipolar usually tend to either have a lot on their plate – leaving little time for reading; or, they just don't feel like doing anything, like reading a lengthy book.

I may quote things said by people who have helped me on my journey; I will not use their names (or real names) for consideration of privacy.

In the following pages; I will share personal experience and things I have learned from therapists and others struggling with Bipolar.

The book is organized in the following way:

First – What is bipolar and what it is not.

Second – What different aspects of bipolar mean for the person who has it; how it can affect a person and their moods. And what I've learned about it.

Third – How it affects me; how I have been treated for it; and how I deal with it.

Fourth – Helpful resources.

Let's get started!

I was diagnosed with severe depression a few times before the doctors finally decided to test me for Bipolar. In 2003, they didn't know as much about it as they do now, but they certainly knew more than when my biological grandmother had it in the mid to late 1900's.

Two things people who have Bipolar need to know – you are not alone and - to be aware of how Bipolar affects you.

Three things that are very hard for people who have Bipolar: to be honest with themselves; understanding they are not defective; and, to forgive themselves for the pain they have caused others because of their symptoms.

I wish to point out that until you understand Bipolar Disorder and how it affects you (or your loved one); it is probably advisable to not speak too freely about it. There is still a stigma attached to mental illness in this country; it is not as bad as it used to be. This will reduce the possibility of misinterpreting, the spread of potential misinformation, and the potential by others to misunderstand you. Again, I urge you to try to refrain from speaking openly about Bipolar Disorder until you understand it well. (which comes from counseling and being treated for it.)

Part 1:

It is my understanding that bipolar is a mental condition due to chemical imbalances in the brain that do not function ‘normally’. It brings on mood swings, with cycles that can range in time from hours to months. For me, it also means that I am hypersensitive to emotional triggers. It doesn’t mean that I am broken or defective.

Bipolar Disorder is a chemical imbalance that affects the frontal lobe of the brain. As my counselor explained it to me: “The pre-frontal lobe is responsible for insight, hindsight, and foresight.”

I also understand that Bipolar is manageable. It can be treated in various ways and the most successful way to make the mood swings and extremes manageable is to treat with medication, counseling and behavior modifications. (I’ll address each separately)

Bipolar has a genetic component; it also has a trauma component. I learned early in my therapy that bipolar can be triggered by a traumatic experience. And that it is typically triggered during the teen years, but not always. Sometimes it becomes apparent in children or does not surface until adulthood.

Bipolar Disorder is also categorized by type. Those types are: Bipolar 1, Bipolar 2, Cyclothymic, Mixed Features, and Rapid-cycling.

The first one includes severe mood episodes that range from mania to depression.

The second one is considered a milder form of Bipolar 1.

The third is described similarly to Bipolar 2, but with shorter episodes.

Mixed Features include simultaneous episodes of mania and depression; racing thoughts and lack of sleep are prevalent in this version.

Rapid-cycling Bipolar is described as having 4 or more episodes within 12 months. (I looked it up on WebMD; although other medical sites can also explain the differences.)

I had many periods of ups and downs in high school and early adulthood. I made many unhealthy decisions: who I spent time with, where I would socialize, and other things. I didn't think much of it because I thought I was unworthy to be happy or to have healthy friends (side effect on the self- confidence from being bullied throughout elementary and junior high school). I thought if I did everything I could to make others happy; even if it meant sacrificing my own health (mental or otherwise), that would make me a good person and other people would like me.

But, eventually, I married and had a child. Instead of worrying about people liking me or making others happy, I focused on being a good mom. That was important to me. For the most part; I did well. But, there were times – in the darkest places of my Bipolar cycle - that I was not making decisions like a good mom; or a good wife.

Sometimes people who have Bipolar get so caught up in their own mood changes that there isn't room for thinking about others… despite the tendency of bipolar people to be nurturing.

When or if this happens to you; don't feel bad or think you are being selfish. People who have Bipolar sometimes need to take care of themselves first. If you aren't your best, how can you give your best to your loved ones?

So, it's 2003; I finally get properly diagnosed as being bipolar. I started on medications – an antidepressant and an anti-manic medicine. We had to try a couple different ones before we found one that seemed to work but didn't make me feel weird.

The first step to being treated for bipolar disorder is to be diagnosed properly. The next step is accepting the diagnosis and the fact that you will be taking at least one medication for the rest of your life.

That second part was hard for me because I had always been anti-drug. I have never been drunk, stoned, or in any other way; high, in my life. I never saw the point in screwing up your brain. We'll get into that a little later.

I also saw a counselor weekly. The counselor helped me with the other parts of treatment – learning about Bipolar, how it affects me, and how to change some things in my everyday life that can help me understand, be aware of, and manage the mood changes. I should note that when I refer to "my Bipolar"; what I mean is how it affects me personally – which may be similar and/or different in the way it affects you or in the symptoms you have.

Part 2

I'll break down the aspects of my treatment in the following pages.

First, the medication. I had to understand the difference between prescribed and properly taken medication and self-medicating (that ineffective method of consuming alcohol, pot, and other drugs that people use to escape their problems).

I have always been against consuming drugs and alcohol to escape problems. I also detested the idea of having to take drugs every day. I had to realize that this would not label me as a druggie, and that the medication I was taking was necessary for my mental health.

Once I understood the difference and realized that me taking medication every day for the rest of my life wasn't really a bad thing because it kept me out of those dark places that the bipolar mind goes when it isn't being treated... most of you; if not all – know what I'm talking about when I say 'dark places'.

Taking my Bipolar medication daily doesn't make me an addict; it makes me wise – because I know it is part of what's helping my moods to stay relatively stable and keeps many of the negative thoughts away.

Here's a tip that I learned – remember that not all medications work for all people. Work with your doctor and be honest about how the medications make you feel so that adjustments can be made until you find the right one/ones.

It is important to note here that it can take up to a year to find the right medication or combination of medications that work for you.

Another tip that I learned – medication isn't supposed to make it go away. It is supposed to reduce the intensity of the moods so that they are at a level you can consciously manage. This can help you handle the mood – so it doesn't affect your daily life and relationships; or doesn't affect your daily life as much.

It is critically important for me to take my medications regularly - daily, as prescribed – so that the extremes of my bipolar mood changes are reduced to a manageable level. I now enjoy life more than I did before I was properly diagnosed and on the right medication.

I urge you to NOT STOP taking medication just because you feel better; the medication is part of what is helping you to feel better!

Second, the counseling. Again, I had to change my way of thinking and understand that just because I had to see a counselor it didn't mean I was broken or defective. Wise people know when to ask for help; and, I knew I needed counseling to help me with my newly diagnosed condition. She helped me a lot, by teaching me about Bipolar Disorder and how it affects me.

The depression was the obvious part; I sought treatment previously – for when I was depressed. So, I was only treated for depression during those previous trips to the doctor. The manic mood was another story. I had heard of "manic-depression" before; but, like most young adults, I thought it only happened to other people; so I didn't pay much attention to it – until it *did* happen to me.

My first counselor said that “manic” means an ‘elevated state of emotion’; however a manic phase has many different faces. It can manifest itself in various ways; and, I would guess that no two people are exactly the same.

It is my understanding, too; that manic manifestations: the elevated state of emotion can be emotions like joy, anger, irritability or more extreme versions like rage, euphoria, and quick irritability.

Mania can also include compulsive behaviors like compulsive shopping or Obsessive Compulsive Disorder. It can include paranoia, anxiety, panic attacks, megalomania, and other such moods. Also, mania tends to make it hard to sleep because the brain keeps running like a hamster on a wheel, even when you are trying to rest. I would try to tell my brain to shut up, but it wouldn’t listen… until I was on anti-manic medicine.

It needs to be said; that even for an individual, manic phases don't always include the same manifestations in every cycle. Sometimes I get irritable mixed with joy. Sometimes I get joy with creative energy. Sometimes I am just grumpy with no other symptoms. In other words; your mania can manifest as any single or combination of your manifestations.

I also learned that Bipolar isn't just a cycle that comes and goes on its own; it can be triggered as well - just as people who don't have Bipolar Disorder can experience something that changes their mood. The difference, I noticed, is that people who have Bipolar Disorder have a hypersensitivity to those mood triggers. It takes much less to cause a mood swing in a person with Bipolar than in a person that does not have it.

Here is a tip I learned – the anti-manic medication could make you drowsy; so try to schedule taking it within an hour or so of your usual bedtime. That way, it can help you fall asleep and still be through your system long enough that you can wake up when you are scheduled to.

Another thing I learned in counseling was that I had to acknowledge the effects it has on me; know that it is my responsibility to deal with those effects – no one can do it for me. I also needed to apologize to loved ones and forgive myself for things I put them through before I was under proper treatment.

If you don't forgive yourself and make peace with loved ones; it makes it hard to move forward, even when being treated.

My counseling also made me aware of some things that most people who have Bipolar have in common are: they tend to be nurturing people, always wanting to help someone; they tend to cling to things of the past at some time in their cycles – sometimes reaching out to people they knew years before or keeping a clutter of things they feel sentimental about.

Many individuals who have Bipolar Disorder also tend to be seen as 'control freaks' by others. But this is necessary – there is nothing wrong with trying to maintain control over aspects of your life that you can actually control. What we can't control is our brain chemistry.

Behavior modification (for lack of a better term) – I refer to the things that I did to help reduce the possibility of mood swings and give me a sense of control. (By the way, all of these topics are good to discuss and help loved ones become aware of; this is important – because loved ones can help you with these)

Topics to discuss are:

1) Having a realistic sense of how my day is going to go – because surprises or sudden changes can throw a bipolar person off or even cause a mood swing.
2) Having morning /bedtime ritual/routine. This can also help bipolar people stay focused and secure in their stability.
3) Planning ahead for anything different than your routine.
4) Personally, I have to plan to put aside time to be spontaneous; I can't just 'be' spontaneous.
5) Schedule chores and activities on a regular basis so you know when to expect to do them.

6) When something unexpected does happen; try to stay calm and think it through. It might not be as bad as it feels. Sometimes it is, sometimes it isn't.
7) Talk with loved ones about your habits and routines so that they understand why routines are necessary for you; and why it could be bad if they upset your routines. They should also understand why you need the sense of control that realistic expectations and habits give you.
8) Explain to loved ones to be on alert for signs of your mood changes, so that they know how you might act during one of your phases or phase changes. This can reduce potential arguments, anxiety, or other forms of stress and tension.

Part 3

Just a reminder; I am not a medical professional, this is not a medical paper or a diagnostic tool; this is my experience and understanding of bipolar – derived from what I have learned and lived through. My experiences may be different than someone else's; and some things may be the same or similar.

All opinions and comments are based on my own experiences; and may not apply to someone else who has been diagnosed as having Bipolar. That being said, I'll continue with how I personally have learned to live with and manage Bipolar.

But first, I want to stress the importance of being correctly diagnosed. I have a friend who was recently diagnosed with Bipolar Disorder. This friend had previously been diagnosed with a variety of other things during the teens years:

Anger issues, ADHD, ADD, Depression, and other things.

Each diagnosis individually made sense. But the medications and counseling for those didn't help much.

This person struggled academically, at work, and sometimes socially. However, recently; someone thought to consider all those symptoms as a whole and he was finally diagnosed with Bipolar Disorder. Thus, he is finally being treated for it.

He indicated to me that the medicine, counseling, and having someone to talk to who knows what it's like; has helped him get better control over aspects of his life that previously alluded him.

He has been able to hold down a job and is better able to control his temper than he used to. This means there is less conflict and potential violence in his life. And that can only be a good thing☺ I'm happy for him.

I learned from reading and counseling; people with ADHD are often misdiagnosed as Bipolar and vice versa; so make sure you tell your doctor anything that might be helpful in determining which of these you may have.

One primary difference is that Bipolar Disorder mostly affects your mood. ADHD mostly affects attention and behavior.

Another difference is that people with Bipolar Disorder have cycles of their moods. Those cycles include depression and hypomania. People with ADHD don't experience the cycling like people with Bipolar do.

It is important to also note that there are symptoms of ADHD and Bipolar that are similar; including: being impulsive, excessive physical energy, and inability to focus or pay attention.

Now: Me and 'my Bipolar' – this is how I live with it: Routines and behavior modification; medication, counseling, family education and adjustment.

I developed an everyday awareness, routines, and reasonable expectations of what will happen during my day. Those three things are big factors that I can do to be able to handle and manage my Bipolar.

I wake up and do my morning routine, then head to work. At work, I know the specifics can vary; but, my duties are pretty much consistent. This is helpful in trying to stay focused when my mind may otherwise wish to wander.

If I have chores to do or errands to run – whether I'm working that day or not - I make a list and label them in the order I want to do them. I make lists a lot; it helps me remember things when my manic brain sometimes goes off in all directions at once.

I conscientiously try to compliment one person each day. Being positive and sharing a positive comment with someone helps me with seeing the bright side of things and with staying positive. I figured, if I can train my brain to default to positive thinking instead of recalling the negative stuff; well – it certainly can't hurt and it might help me maintain control over at least some of my mood changes. And indeed, it does seem to. This may not work for everyone; but, as difficult as it can be; it's worth a try.

Let me give an example of how this default to positive thinking over negative thinking helped me with a stressor one morning.

I woke up as usual. My routine at the time included running my child and some of his friends to school before I headed into work. When we were getting ready to leave, I realized I could not find my keys.

This could have upset me and messed with my moods; but... in my efforts to think positive - first I remained calm enough to handle each problem caused by my losing my keys – one thing at a time.

First, the kids; I contacted one of the kids' grandparents (as that was who he was being raised by) to see if the grandparent could take the kids to school, just for this morning... the grandparent said yes. One problem solved.

Next, where did I remembering having my keys last? The grocery store. My options were to call spouse or my parents (who usually kept a spare key to my car in case they have to borrow it).

The spouse was at work and to have him miss work to take me to grocery store to see if they had my keys might get him in trouble.

My dad, he forgets and loses things semi-regularly too; so, he would not be annoyed with me if I asked him for help. (This was before cell phones were so widely spread and smart phones definitely didn't exist yet; so I used a land line to make the call.)

So, I called my dad, then, I called work, to say why I was running a little bit late. My dad arrived and took me to grocery store. We got my keys from the store and he dropped me back at home; and I went to work… no problem.

In this circumstance, I was able to control my mood on some level so I could work through the problems caused by my losing my keys – rather than getting upset, frustrated and causing my mood to become negative.

Another example: same situation; but I called my spouse instead of my dad. My spouse would have probably scolded me for not keeping better track of my keys, especially since it could have gotten him in trouble at work for having to leave when he wasn't on lunch. This would have caused my mood to sour and I would not have been able to change it. I would have likely had a foul day for the whole day.

Sometimes we can have some control over our moods, mood triggers, and mood changes; and break the feeling of being in a downward spiral. Sometimes, we can't.

But unless we learn and acknowledge what the symptoms are for our own mood changes; *and* recognize what manifestations of a cycle we are currently experiencing; we will have little success in calming ourselves to handle it without destabilizing.

The medicine is another key factor in my managing my Bipolar. It's absolutely necessary to keep taking the medication, once you and your doctor found medications that work for you. I adjusted the time I take my medication so that it is in line with the times I usually wake up for work and go to bed at night.

I do this because the anti-manic medication makes me drowsy. It usually takes anywhere between 30 minutes and a couple hours before I get drowsy; so I make sure I take it about an hour before I plan to go to bed.

It is also important that any and all of the doctors you see – regardless of the reason you see them - know about the medication you take for bipolar. And, whether you see a psychiatrist or family doctor for your prescriptions, always tell them how the medication is working for you and if you are having any side effect. Also tell them if it makes you feel off or odd in any way.

If that doctor isn't listening to you or taking your observations into consideration; find another doctor. It's your health, your body; you have a right to say you want a different doctor because – for whatever reason – you don't like the one you have.

Which brings me to my next point regarding managing my own bipolar, a counselor – it's important to have one that listens to you and interacts with you; not one that just listens and takes notes.

Currently, I have a therapist that has a field specialization in Bipolar. When I was first diagnosed with Bipolar there weren't specialized counselors in my area. By having specializations in the counseling field indicates to me; that they are learning more about the conditions and illnesses that need counseling as part of the treatment of those conditions.

In my experience; there are things that a good counselor does and doesn't do. They do not judge or criticize. Nor do they take notes and remain silent.

They <u>do</u> listen, offer clarifications, provide suggestions based on their professional knowledge, and help their patient learn about symptoms of Bipolar; and discover which symptoms the patient experiences.

If you always leave your counselor's office feeling worse than before you went; consider why you feel worse. If it is because the counselor is being judgmental, critical, or negative; seek a different counselor. It is your right as a patient.

I'm glad that we (collectively as a society and the collective of professionals) continue to pursue information about conditions like Bipolar Disorder. The more we know, the better we can treat ourselves.

Something we didn't know about Bipolar Disorder when I was first diagnosed; but learned later; is that the intensity, level, fluctuations of Bipolar only increase as one ages. This is something to keep in mind so you can be aware of such changes because it could mean you should modify your medication.

Of course, teaching my family about Bipolar and my own version of it helps them understand it. That understanding is what let them decide how to accommodate me.

They know not to surprise me; not even a good surprise. They know to be patient with me when I sometimes get jumbled in thoughts when I talk. They know to not take my need to control some things personally. They know to ask or tell me ahead of time of things that might change an event in some way… like inviting someone unexpected to a holiday gathering, or for Sunday brunch.

Having Bipolar and understanding that I have to sometimes put myself and my mental health first isn't being selfish. Because if we ignore our symptoms, stop taking medication, don't talk to others, and just stumble along Bipolar's uneven path; we will continue to make decisions that can negatively affect us and our loved ones.

Sometimes; putting myself first means I have to let go of friendships or steer away from acquaintances that are unstable or destabilizing.

I want to relay a situation that another person (we'll call John) with Bipolar had told to me. John had a friend (we'll call Linda) that was mostly fun to be around, but, had a sporadic personality. Linda frequently acted and reacted spontaneously and randomly. Linda was unpredictable.

I know that I can't be spontaneous; I need structure and for things to be planned out. John is much the same way; so he had trouble being around Linda.

Linda wasn't consistent about anything. The bottom line was that Linda's presence caused John a lot of instability, worry, and anxiety. So, I suggested that he reduced the amount of time he spent around Linda. To my knowledge, they eventually stopped communicating.

I would have done the same thing because people who do or say things that make me feel like the ground is being pulled out from under me, and throw my mood out of whack are bad for me. This is true for people with bipolar. It's an instant feeling of losing control and feeling destabilized. To be honest, I don't like it and I don't handle it well. Neither did John. He was less stressed after distancing himself from Linda.

John's options were to either change himself or the situation. In this case, the situation was easier to modify. He took my advice and chose to distance himself from Linda, in order to keep some control over his stability.

It is important for people who have Bipolar to stay away or get out of relationships that destabilize them; no matter how nice the person can be or how much you like that person when they aren't destabilizing you.

I want to point out, I have been told in counseling that persons who have Bipolar tend to have difficulties with relationships and sometimes. They may find it easier to move from one relationship to another instead fixing it. I'm glad I chose to work on the relationships that bring me stability and stay away from ones that don't.

For me, personally; I need to have stable friendships; and, not ones that throw me off balance.

The up side... yes; there can be an upside to bipolar – usually comes during my manic phase; it's called 'creative energy'. I don't get creative energy in every manic phase. I'd say I get that energy in about 60% of my manic episodes.

It is my understanding that people who have Bipolar; in addition to things like being nurturing and sentimental; also can be very artistic. For me; it's mostly writing. I get other creative ideas too; but writing has been the primary medium for harnessing my creative energy.

I have a couple of poetry collections that have been published recently. In each of those collections, there is a poem about bipolar. I will share two of them in this book too.

This first one is reflective on how I saw myself when I first was diagnosed. It is called “Rapidfire Misfire”.

Cascading mass of thoughts and feelings;
amid endlessly swirling chaos,
and the train of thought that never stops…
not even for a moment.
Waking; feeling weary,
Bewildered, and exhausted.
Wanting to sleep the day away,
But unable to find a quiet place in my head.
Apathy and compassion hasten their intricate dance
On a battlefield of rambling disconnect and rapid misfires.
Internal combat scars the defective brain;
Always struggling to not destabilize.
Lurking beneath the mask of steel,
Lies the flawed mind; aspiring for normal,
Always reaching, but never achieving...
Broken mind; broken spirit…

This second one is reflective of the general struggle with bipolar; (I am working on a poem about successfully living with it too; it's still in early stages). This one is simply called, "Bipolar".

Strings of thought whirl about

Where sense and logic have no place

One by one, building a cage

Around my mind; I can't escape.

This beverage of bipolar;

Manic with a depression chaser...

Random compulsions

A mental circuit breaker

Cargo of joy, fear, rage, impatience

Life's unexpected takes its toll...

Limitless emotions ramble recklessly,

Along this misguided road

A sudden shift surfaces;

Fissure opens & thoughts explode.

Hijacked emotions, cascade outward

Security and reason; I cannot hold.

Floating in murky seas of instability

Irrational isolation & wandering lost;

Always wondering what is real

And what is not...

I'm not a visual artist; I can barely draw stick figures. I hope that whatever artistic gift you have; visual art, reading stories, writing poems, singing, dancing, playing an instrument, or whatever it is that you do; please keep doing it.

Consider sharing your gift with others. And if you find yourself procrastinating to complete those things; when manic comes around again – use it to do something positive.

In summary:

1) Once diagnosed; accept it so you can move onto treatment.
2) Learn about Bipolar Disorder and its symptoms
3) Seek a counselor that can help teach you and guide you with your symptoms and mood swings. more about it with techniques to help you manage it
4) Learn and understand how it manifests in you and in your life
5) Seek a doctor that can help you find the right medication or combination of medications that help you as an individual with Bipolar Disorder. Then, once you find that combination, do not stop taking them.
6) Modify your daily life to include routines and habits. This can help you achieve a sense of control over some aspects of your life and give you a sense of stability.
7) Share the process with your loved ones; as they can be helpful through some parts of treatment and healing.

8) Don't punish yourself nor forget to forgive yourself, especially when others have already forgiven you.
9) Remember; the intensity (and potential fluctuation) of Bipolar Disorder only increases with age. Sometimes it increases a lot; in other people, it is barely noticeable. In order to manage that increased intensity or increased fluctuation; you have to be aware that it could be happening. Managing that increase could mean modifying your medication, increasing your counseling sessions, or more regular habits.

I hope this book helps you understand and define Bipolar; don't let Bipolar define you.

While I tried to include the basics in this short book; there is more information out there that might be helpful. So, I'm including some resources for bipolar people:

https://www.samhsa.gov/find-help/disorders

https://www.nimh.nih.gov/health/publications/bipolar-disorder-listing.shtml

https://www.webmd.com/bipolar-disorder/guide/bipolar-disorder-resources-1

https://www.dbsalliance.org/support/chapters-and-support-groups/

*I have come across the sites while researching online but have not actually used any of them. However, my counseling sessions are very helpful. I included the sites above, in case you want to look at them to see if they offer more insight than what you currently have.

Thank you for reading my book; I sincerely hope it helps you.

If you like poetry, or like the poems I included in this book; please check out my other books:

Love, Life, and Spirit – A Collection of Poetry.

Mind, Heart, and Soul – A Collection of Poetry.

Both available on Amazon, or email me: for information on where to get copies of my books, signing events, and on upcoming 2020 releases.

cmalky@hotmail.com

www.ingramcontent.com/pod-product-compliance
Lightning Source LLC
Chambersburg PA
CBHW051430250726
48656CB00020B/2186

* 9 7 8 1 7 0 3 6 0 5 4 4 0 *